YOGA ANATOMY KEYS

The Functional Guide for Beginners

By

Holly Emily Walker

DISCLAIMER

This document is geared towards providing exact and suitable information in regards to the topic and issue covered in this book. The publication is sold on the concept that the publisher is not required to render an accounting, officially allowed, or otherwise qualified service. If advice is necessary, legal or professionals, a practiced individual in the profession should be called.

From a Declaration of Principles that was accepted and approved equally by a Committee of the American Bar Association and a Committee of Publishers and Associations.

In no way is it legal to reproduce, duplicate, from, or transmit any part of this document by either a printed format or electronic means. Recording of this publication is highly prohibited, and any storage of this document is not allowed unless with written permission from the publisher. All rights reserved.

The information provided herein is stated to be truthful and consistent, in that any liability, in terms of inattention or otherwise, by any usage or abuse of any policies, processes, or directions contained within is the solitary and utter responsibility of the recipient reader. Under no circumstances will any legal responsibility or blame be held against the publisher for any reparation, damages, or monetary loss due to the information herein, either directly or indirectly.

The respective author owns all copyrights not held by the publisher.

The information herein is offered for informational purposes solely and is universal as so.

The presentation of the information is without a contract or any type of guarantee assurance.

The trademarks that are used are without any consent, and the publication of the trademark is without permission or backing by the trademark owner. All trademarks and brands within this book are for clarifying purposes only and are owned by the owners themselves, not affiliated with this document.

TABLE OF CONTENTS

Introduction

Yoga is now regarded in the Western world as a holistic approach to health and is classified by the National Institutes of Health as a form of Complementary and Alternative Medicine (CAM). The word "Yoga" comes from a Sanskrit root "Yuj," which means union, it direct and concentrate one's attention. The regular practice of yoga promotes strength, endurance, flexibility, and facilitates characteristics of friendliness, compassion, and greater self-control while cultivating a sense of calmness and well-being. The result of continuous yoga practice leads to changes in life perspective, self-awareness, and an improved understanding of energy to live life fully and with genuine enjoyment. The constant practice of yoga produces a physiological state opposite to that of the fight stress response, and with that interruption in the stress response, a sense of balance and union between the mind and body will be achieved.

Yoga is a form of mind-body fitness that involves the combination of muscular activity while an internally directed mindful focus on awareness of the self, the breath, and energy. Four basic principles control the teachings and practices of yoga's healing system.

The first principle is the human body, which is a holistic entity comprised of various interrelated dimensions that are not separable from one another while the health or illness of any of this dimension affects the other aspects.

The second principle is individuals and their needs, which are different and must be approached in a way that acknowledges this individuality.

The third principle is yoga is self-empowering; the student is his or her healer. Yoga engages the student in the healing process, the students an active role in their journey toward their health, the healing comes from within, instead of from an outside source.

The fourth principle is that the quality and state of an individual's mind. The mind of an individual is crucial to healing. When the individual has positive mind-state healing happens more quickly, whereas if the mind-state is negative, healing may be prolonged.

Patanjali first described yoga philosophy and practice in the classic text, *Yoga Sutras*, which is widely acknowledged as the authoritative text on yoga. Today, many people identify yoga by the physical practice of Yoga (asana), but asana is just one of the many tools used for healing the individual; only three of the 196 sutras mention asana, and the remainder of the text discusses the other components of yoga including conscious breathing, meditation, lifestyle and diet changes, visualization and the use of sound, among many others

The eight limbs are comprised of ethical principles for living a meaningful and purposeful life, serving as a prescription for moral and ethical conduct and self-discipline; they direct attention towards one's health while acknowledging the spiritual aspects of one's nature. Any of the eight limbs may be used separately, but within yoga philosophy, the physical postures and breathing exercises prepare the mind and body for meditation and spiritual development. Based on Patanjali's eight limbs, many different yogic disciplines have been developed. Each has its technique for preventing and treating disease. The most common aspects of yoga practiced are the physical postures and breathing practices of Hatha Yoga and meditation.

Hatha yoga enhances the capacity of the physical body through the use of a series of body postures, movements (asanas), and breathing techniques (pranayama). The breathing techniques of Hatha yoga focus on the conscious prolongation of inhalation, breathe retention, and exhalation. It is through the consolidation of the physical body and breath while performing the postures and movements that blockages in the energy channels of the body are cleared, and the body energy system becomes more balanced. Although numerous styles of Hatha Yoga exist, the majority of studies included in this manuscript utilized the Iyengar style of yoga. The Iyengar method of Hatha Yoga is based on the teachings of the yoga master B.K.S. Iyengar. Iyengar yoga places emphasis on standing poses to develop strength, stability, stamina, concentration, and body alignment. Props are utilized to facilitate learning and to adjust poses, and instruction is given on how to use yoga to ease various ailments and stressors.

Yoga is recognized as a form of mind-body medicine that integrates an individual's physical, mental, and spiritual components to improve aspects of health, mainly stress-related illnesses. The evidence shows that stress contributes to the diagnosis of heart disease, cancer, and stroke as well as other chronic conditions and diseases. Since stress is implicated in numerous diseases, it is a priority to include a focus on stress management and reduction of negative emotional states to reduce the burden of illness. Viewed as a holistic stress management technique, yoga is a form of CAM (Complementary and Alternative Medicine) that produces a physiological sequence of events in the body, reducing the stress response. The scientific study of yoga has increased extensively in recent years, and many clinical trials have been designed to assess its therapeutic effects and benefits.

Chapter 1 - Introduction To Yoga

Yoga is a spiritual discipline based on a degree of subtle science, which focuses on bringing agreement between mind and body. Yoga is an art and science of healthy living. The word 'Yoga' is derived from the Sanskrit root 'Yuj,' which means 'to join' or 'to yoke' or 'to unite.' As per Yogic scriptures, the practice of yoga leads to the union of individual consciousness with that of the universal consciousness, indicating a perfect agreement between the mind and body. According to modern scientists believes, everything which exists in the universe is just a manifestation of the same quantum firmament. Someone who experiences this oneness of existence is known to be in yoga, having attained to a state of freedom referred to as mukti, nirvana, or moksha. Thus the aim of Yoga is Self-realization, to overcome all kinds of sufferings leading to 'the state of liberation' (Moksha) or 'freedom' (Kaivalya).

Living with freedom from all walks of life, health and harmony shall be the main objectives of Yoga practice. "Yoga" also refers to fundamental science that is made up of diverse methods through which human beings can actualize this union and have dominion over their destiny. Yoga, being widely considered as an 'immortal cultural outcome' of Indus Saraswati Valley civilization – dating back to 2700 B.C., has proved itself to approve both material and spiritual upliftment of humanity. Fundamental human values are very similar to Yoga Sadhana.

A Brief History and Development of Yoga

Yoga practice is believed to have started since the beginning of civilization. It is thought that the science of yoga has its source thousands of years ago, long before any religions or belief systems were born. In the yogic lore, Shiva is seen as the first yogi or Adiyogi, and the first Guru or Adi Guru.

Thousand years ago, on the banks of the lake Kantisarovar in the Himalayas, Adiyogi discharged his profound knowledge into a legendary called Saptarishis or "Seven Sages." The sages transmit this robust yogic science to different parts of the world, including Asia, Northern Africa, the Middle East, and South America. Interestingly, modern scholars have noted and wondered at the close parallels found between ancient cultures across the globe. However, it was in India that the yogic system found its fullest expression. Agastya, the Saptarishi who traveled across the Indian subcontinent, crafted this culture around a core Yogic way of life.

Yogic motives and figures performing Yoga Sadhana suggest the presence of yoga in ancient India. The phallic symbols seals of the idols of mother Goddess are suggestive of Tantra Yoga. Presence of Yoga is available in folk traditions, Indus valley civilization, Vedic and Upanishadic heritage, Buddhist and Jain traditions, Darshanas, epics of Mahabharat and Ramayana, theistic legends of Shaivas, Vaishnavas, and Tantric traditions. Also, there was a pure Yoga, which has been manifested in the mystical traditions of South Asia.

During this time, yoga had to be rehearsal under the direct guidance of Guru, and its spiritual value was given particular importance. It was a part of Upasana, and yoga sadhana was inbuilt in their rituals. The highest emphasis during the Vedic period was given to the sun. This affects the practice of 'Surya Namaskar' may have been invented then. Pranayama was a part of daily ritual and to offer the oblation. Though yoga was being practiced in the pre-Vedic season, the great Sage Maharshi Patanjali arranged it into a systematic order and codified the then existing practices of yoga. After Patanjali, many Sages and Yoga Masters contributed significantly to the preservation and development of yoga practices through their well-documented practices and literature.

Before the Vedic period (2700 B.C.), the historical pieces of evidence of the existence of yoga was found and after that till Patanjali's period. The primary sources in which we get almost all the information about Yoga practices and the related literature during this period are available in Vedas (4), Upanishads (108), Smritis, teachings of Buddhism, Jainism, Panini, Epics (2), Puranas (18), etc.

Tentatively, the period between 500 BC and 800 A.D. is considered as the Classical period, which is also considered as the most productive and prominent period in the history and development of yoga. During this period, expositions of Vyasa on Yoga Sutras and Bhagavadgita, etc., came into existence. The two great religious teachers of India –Mahavir and Buddha performs a significant role in the commentary of Vyasa on Yoga Sutras. The concept of five great vows – Pancha mahavrata- by Mahavir and Ashta Magga or eightfold path by Buddha may be well reflected on as primitive nature of Yoga sadhana. We find its more explicit explanation in Bhagavadgita, which has elaborately presented the concept of Gyan yoga, Bhakti yoga, and Karma Yoga. These three types of yoga are still the highest example of human wisdom, and even till today, people find peace by following the methods as shown in Gita. Patanjali's yoga sutra, besides containing various aspects of yoga, is mainly identified with the eightfold path of yoga. The critical commentary on Yoga sutra by Vyasa was also written.

During this particular time, the aspect of mind was given prominence, and it was brought out through Yoga sadhana. Mind and body both can be brought under control to experience calmness. The period between 800 A.D. - 1700 A.D. has been recognized as the Post Classical period wherein the teachings of great Acharyatrayas-Adi Shankracharya, Ramanujacharya, and Madhavacharya- were prominent during this period. The lessons of Suradasa, Tulasidasa, Purandardasa, Mirabai were great contributors during this period. The Natha Yogis of Hathayoga Tradition like Matsyendaranatha, Gorkshanatha, Cauranginatha, Swatmaram Suri, Gheranda, Shrinivasa Bhatt are some of the selfless minds who popularized the Hatha Yoga practices during this period.

The period between 1700 and 1900 A.D. is observed as the Modern period in which the great Yogacharyas- Ramana Maharshi, Ramakrishna Paramhansa, Paramhansa Yogananda, Vivekananda, etc., have contributed to the development of Raja Yoga. This was the period when Vedanta, Bhakti yoga, Nathayoga, or Hatha-yoga flourished. The Shadanga-yoga of Gorakshashatakam, Chaturanga-yoga of Hathayogapradipika, Saptanga-yoga of Gheranda Samhita, were the central tenents of Hatha-yoga.

Now in contemporary times, everybody has a conviction about yoga practices towards the preservation, maintenance, and promotion of health. Yoga has spread all over the world through the teachings of great personalities like Swami Shivananda, Shri T.Krishnamacharya, Swami Kuvalayananda, Shri Yogendra, Swami Rama, Sri Aurobindo, Maharshi Mahesh Yogi, Acharya Rajanish, Pattabhi Jois, B.K.S. Iyengar, Swami Satyananda Sarasvati, and the likes.

For many people, the practice of yoga is restricted to Hatha Yoga and Asanas (Postures). However, among the Yoga Sutras, just three sutras are dedicated to asanas.

Hatha yoga is a preparatory process so that the body can sustain higher levels of energy. The process begins with the body, then the breath, the mind, and the inner self.

Yoga has also been generally accepted as a therapy or exercise system for health and fitness. While the physical and mental health is the natural consequences of yoga, the purpose of yoga is more far-reaching. "Yoga is about an agreement between oneself with the universe. It is the technology of aligning individual geometry about the universe, to achieve the highest level of perception and harmony."

Yoga does cleave to any particular religion, community, or belief system; it has always been approached as a technology for inner well-being. Anyone who practices yoga with involvement can obtain its benefits, irrespective of the person's faith, ethnicity, or culture.

Traditional Schools of Yoga

These different Philosophies, culture, lineages, race, and Guru-shishya paramparas of yoga lead to the appearances of several Traditional Schools of Yoga, e.g., Jnana-yoga, Bhakti-yoga, Karma-yoga, Dhyana-yoga, Patanjala-yoga, Kundalini-yoga, Hatha-yoga, Mantra-yoga, Laya-yoga, Raja-yoga, Jain-yoga, Bouddha-yoga, etc. Each school has its practices and principles towards achieving the goals of yoga.

Yogic Practices for Health and Wellness

Yoga Sadhanas is widely practiced by Yama, Niyama, Asana, Pranayama, Pratyahara, Dharana, Dhyana (Meditation), Samadhi/Samyama, Bandhas & Mudras, Shat-karmas, Yukta-Sahara, Yukta karma, Mantra Japa, etc. Yama's are restraints, and Niyama's are governed by a rule. These are considered to be pre-requisites for the Yoga Sadhanas (Practices). Asanas can achieve stability of the body and mind "Kuryat-tad-asanam-sthairyam," comprise in adopting diverse body (psycho-physical) patterns, giving the ability to maintain a particular body position for a significant period.

The developing consciousness of one's breathing, followed by voluntary regulation of respiration as the functional basis of one's existence, is known as pranayama. Pranayama helps in developing knowledge of one's mind, and it also helps to establish control over the same account. This is done by promoting awareness of the 'flow of in-breath and out-breath' (svasa-prasvasa) through nostrils, mouth, and other body openings, its interior and exterior pathways. Later, this event is modified, through regulated principles and controlled, leading to the awareness of the body spaces getting filled (puraka); the spaces remaining in a populated state are getting emptied (rechaka) during the period it has been regulated and controlled.

The separation of one's consciousness (withdrawal) from the sense organs is indicated by Pratyahara, which helps one to remain connected with the external objects. The field attention (inside the body and mind), which is usually understood as concentration is indicated as Dharana. Dhyana (Meditation) is contemplation (focused attention inside the body and mind)

Bandhas and Mudras are viewed as the higher Yogic practices, mainly believes in the adaptation of some particular body (psycho-physical) patterns along with control over respiration. This further helps to preside the control over minds and paves the way for higher yogic attainment. Shat-karmas are de-toxification procedures; help to remove the poisonous stored in the body, and are clinical.

Yuktahara (Right Food and other inputs) is in support of appropriate food and food habits for healthy living. However, the practice of Dhyana (Meditation) helps in self-realization that leads to a level beyond the range of ordinary perception, which has been considered as the essence of Yoga Sadhana (The Practice of Yoga).

The Fundamentals of Yoga Sadhana

Yoga works on the level of one's body, mind, emotion, and energy. With this, yoga can be classified into four broad:

1. Karma yoga; where we exploit the body;
2. Bhakti yoga, where we use the emotions;
3. Gyana yoga, where we utilize the mind and intellect,
4. Kriya yoga; where we use the energy.

Every system of yoga we practice would fall within the range of one or more of these categories. Every individual in the universe is a unique combination of these four factors. "All the ancient facts on Yoga have stressed that it is crucial to function under the guidance of a Guru." It has been believed that only a Guru can mix the apt combination of the four original paths, as it is inevitable for each seeker.

Yoga Education

Traditionally, The Education of Yoga was impacted by knowledgeable, experienced, and wise persons in the families and then by the Seers. Yoga Education, on the other hand, Yoga Education aims at taking care of the individual, the 'Being.' It is presumed that a right, balanced, integrated, truthful, clean, transparent person will be more useful to oneself, family, society, nation, nature, and humanity at large. Yoga education is 'Being oriented.' Details of working with the 'being oriented' aspect have been outlined in various living traditions, and texts and the method contributing to this vital field is known as "Yoga."

Present days, The Education of Yoga is being impacted by many remarkable Yoga Institutions, Yoga Colleges, Yoga Universities, Naturopathy colleges, and Private trusts & societies. Many Yoga Clinics, Yoga Therapy, and Training Centers, Preventive Health Care Units of Yoga, Yoga Research Centers, etc., have been established in Hospitals,

Dispensaries, Medical Institutions, and Therapeutically setups.

Several social customs and rituals in India, the land of yoga, reflect a love for ecological balance, tolerance towards other systems of thought, and a compassionate outlook towards all creations.

Chapter 2 - Meaning Of Yoga

The term "Yoga" originates from a Sanskrit word meaning "Union." The merging of physical exercises, mental meditation, and breathing techniques to strengthen the muscles and relieve stress is known as YOGA.

Yoga practices with the mind and body have a 5,000 years history in ancient Indian philosophy. Yoga styles combine physical postures, breathing techniques, and meditation or relaxation. In more recent years, it has become popular as a form of physical exercise based upon poses that promote improved control of the mind and body and enhance well-being.

The practice of yoga has many disciplines with different types. This chapter explores the philosophy and various branches of yoga.

Philosophy

This helps to relay the spiritual message and guide sessions, and yoga often uses the imagery of a tree with roots, a trunk, branches, blossoms, and fruits. Each "Branch" of yoga represents a different focus and set of characteristics.

The six branches are:

1. **Hatha Yoga**: This deals with the physical and mental department designed to prime the body and mind.
2. **Raja Yoga**: This branch deals with the meditation and strict agreement to a series of disciplinary steps known as the "Eight Limbs" of yoga.
3. **Karma Yoga**: This is a path of service that deals with the desire to create a future free from negativity and selfishness.
4. **Bhakti Yoga**: This aims to create the path of devotion, religion, a positive way to channel emotions and cultivate acceptance and tolerance.
5. **Jnana Yoga**: This branch deals with wisdom, the path of the scholar, which enables them to develop the intellect through study.
6. **Tantra Yoga**: This is a significant pathway of ritual, ceremony, or consummation of a relationship.

The process of approaching yoga with a specific purpose in mind can help an individual decide which branch he/she need to follow.

Chakras

The word "Chakra" literally means the spinning wheel.

Yoga believes that chakras are center points of all energy, thoughts, feelings, and the physical body. Chakras determine the way people experience reality through several means, such as emotional reactions, desires, levels of confidence or fear, and even physical symptoms and effects; yogic teachers have highlighted this,

When physical, mental or emotional imbalances have been triggered, and then there is an energy blockage in the chakra which manifests in symptoms, such as anxiety, lethargy, or poor digestion.

Asanas are the many physical positions in Hatha Yoga. People who practice yoga use asanas to free energy and stimulate an imbalanced chakra.

There are seven major chakras, each with their focus:

1. **Sahasrara**: This can also be referred to as the "Thousand-crown." The state of pure consciousness was represented by chakra. This chakra can be found at the crown of the head, and it has a color white or violet, which describes it. Sahasrara involves matters of inner wisdom and physical death.
2. **Ajna**: This can also be referred to as the "Command" or "Third-eye Chakra" this is a meeting point between two weighty energetic streams in the body. Ajna is similar in colors as violet, indigo, or deep blue, though traditional yoga practitioners describe it as white. The Ajna chakra relates to the hypothesis gland, which drives growth and development.
3. **Vishuddha**: This has a color of red or blue, which represents the "Especially Pure" or Throat" chakra.

Practitioners consider this chakra to be the home of speech, hearing, and metabolism.

4. **Anahata**: This can also be referred to as the "Unstruck" or "Heart." It's related to the colors green and pink. The key issues involving Anahata include complex emotions, compassion, tenderness, unconditional love, equilibrium, rejection, and well-being.

5. **Manipura**: The Yellow color represents the "Jewel City" or "Navel" chakra. Practitioners connect this chakra with the digestive system, and it has been attached as personal power, fear, anxiety, developing opinions, and tendencies towards an introverted personality.

6. **Svadhishthana**: Practitioners claim that the "One's Base" or "Pelvic" chakra is the home of the reproductive organs, the genitourinary system, and the adrenal gland.

7. **Muladhara**: The "Root Support" or "Root Chakra" is at the base of the spine in the coccygeal region. It is said to contain our natural urges relating to food, sleep, sex, and survival as well as the source of avoidance and fear.

Types and Styles of Yoga Include:

Ashtanga Yoga: This type of yoga uses and believes in the ancient yoga teachings. However, it became popular during the 1970s. Ashtanga applies six established sequences of postures that rapidly link every movement to breathe.

Bikram Yoga: This is also referred to as "Hot" yoga. For this process, the room is artificially heated, with temperatures of nearly 105 degrees and 40 percent humidity. It consists of 26 poses and a sequence of two breathing exercises.

Hatha Yoga: This is a general term for any type of yoga that teaches physical postures.

Iyengar Yoga: This type focuses on finding the correct alignment in each pose using a range of props, such as blocks, blankets, straps, chairs, and bolsters.

Kripalu Yoga: This kind of style teaches practitioners to know, accept, and learn from the body. There are several classes a student of Kripalu undergoes. The classes usually begin with breathing exercises and gentle stretches, followed by a series of individual poses and final relaxation.

Kundalini Yoga: This simply means "Coiled, like a snake." Kundalini yoga aims to release pent-up energy.

A class typically begins with chanting and ends with singing. In between, it features asana, pranayama, and meditation customized to create a specific outcome.

Power Yoga: Practitioners have developed this in the year 1980; this based on the traditional ashtanga system.

Sivananda: This is a system based on a five-point philosophy. The philosophy includes breathing, relaxation, diet, exercise, and positive thinking, which work together to form a healthy yogic lifestyle.

Viniyoga: Viniyoga can adapt to any person; it deals with studying the different parts of an organized body regardless of physical ability. Viniyoga teachers require in-depth training and tend to be experts on anatomy and yoga therapy.

Yin: This is a quiet, devotional yoga practice; it is also called Taoist yoga. Yin yoga allows the release of tension in critical joints of the body which including The ankles, knees, hips, the whole back, neck, and the shoulders

Yin poses are passive, meaning that gravity shoulders most of the force and effort.

Prenatal Yoga: this deals with pregnant people. Prenatal yoga uses postures that practitioners have designed for people who are pregnant. It can also support people in getting back into shape after pregnancy as well as promoting health during pregnancy.

Restorative Yoga: This is called the relaxing method of yoga. A person can spend a therapeutic yoga class in four or five simple poses, using props like blankets and bolsters to sink into deep relaxation without exerting any effort in holding the pose.

Yoga classes consist of a set of specific exercises, called poses, combined with specific breathing techniques and meditation principles. If a posture causes pain or proves too difficult, some other variations and modifications can be made to help students. The variety includes props like blocks, blankets, and straps, and even chairs can be used to help you get the most benefit from the poses. Yoga is not one-size-fits-all: Your individual needs and goals will determine the best yoga workout for you.

The benefits of a regular yoga practice are wide-ranging. In general, a complete yoga workout can help keep your back and joints healthy, improve your overall posture, stretch and strengthen muscles and improve your balance, say, Roger Cole, Ph.D., a psycho-biologist and certified Iyengar yoga teacher. Yoga also has "A restorative side that is deeply relaxing and rejuvenating," Dr. Cole says. "Relaxation is built into every yoga session."

Besides, yoga's focus on the breath can calm you and help you learn to be more mindful of your body, says Dr. Timothy McCall, the author of "Yoga as Medicine," and that can help you to move with greater ease.

In recent years, more and more research is demonstrating the wide-ranging health benefits of yoga. Studies show that yoga can help:

Reduce Back Pain: when practicing yoga weekly, it helps to relieve symptoms of low back pains as well as intense, regular stretching sessions.

Strengthen Bones: Yoga practitioners were shown to have increased bone density in their spine and hips, compared to people in a control group.

Improve Balance: Male athletes undergoing yoga training has displayed better balance after ten weeks of yoga classes than a control group of athletes who did not change their routines.

Stave Off Mental Decline: participants who had memory defect, it advisable they do the combination of yoga and meditation as opposed to a brain-training exercise performed much better on a test of visuospatial memory, a type of remembering that is important for balance, depth perception, and the ability to recognize objects and navigate the world.

Reduce Stress: A study of 72 women establish a founding that Iyengar yoga helped reduce mental distress and the related psychological and physical symptoms of anxiety.

Relieve Depression: In a research of coal miners with chronic obstructive pulmonary disease, or C.O.P.D., yoga was shown to alleviate depression and anxiety.

Ancient, But Not Foreign

It is said that yoga is connected to ancient Indian philosophy, so yoga poses have both Sanskrit and English names — *adho mukha svanasana* is more usually known as a downward-facing dog, for example, you may hear both in a class.

Without being in yoga class, even if you have never tried yoga practices, you may already be familiar with some yoga poses. Ever tried a plank? You've done yoga.

There are several trainers and fitness classes around the world, not to mention college and professional sports teams, which includes yoga as a traditional workout with a potent form of mind-body conditioning, helping athletes to breathe better and increase their focus.

It should be noted that many top sports professionals, including the basketball star Lebron James and the tennis champion Novak Djokovic, have incorporated yoga into their training programs.

"The attention-focusing and alignment-honing potential of a yoga practice is a solid complement to more athletic, explosive, and calisthenic endeavors," says Derek Cook, a former personal trainer who teaches yoga.

Risks and Side Effects

Yoga is low-impact and always safe for people when a well-trained instructor is guiding the practice.

Injury due to yoga does not happen frequently and has no barrier to continued practice, and severe damage due to yoga is rare. However, consider a few factors before starting.

Anyone who is pregnant or who has an on-going medical condition, such as high blood pressure, glaucoma, or sciatica, should talk to their healthcare practitioner before practicing yoga. They may need to change or avoid some yoga poses.

Beginners should avoid extreme poses and complicated techniques, such as headstand, lotus position, and forceful breathing.

When using yoga to manage a condition, do not replace conventional medical care with yoga or postpone seeing a healthcare provider about pain or any other medical problem.

Chapter 3 - Benefits Of Yoga

Western science is starting to provide some tangible clues as to how yoga could work to improve health, heal aches and pains, and keep sickness at a laurel. Once you understand them, you'll have even more motivation to step onto your mat, and you probably won't feel so tired to practices more. In the year 2002, I have authentically experienced yoga's healing power. Weeks before a trip to India to investigate yoga therapy, I developed hypoesthesia and tingling in my left hand. After first considering frightening things like a brain tumor and multiple sclerosis, I figured out that the cause of the symptoms was thoracic outlet syndrome, a nerve blockage in my neck, and chest.

Despite the uncomfy symptoms, I realized how useful my condition could be during my trip. While visiting various yoga therapy centers, I would use myself as a specimen for evaluation and treatment by the numerous experts I'd arranged to observe. I could try their suggestions and see if their idea worked for me. While this wasn't exactly a controlled scientific experiment, I knew that such hands-on learning could teach me things I might not otherwise understand.

My experiment proved illuminating. At the Vivekananda ashram just outside of Bangalore, S. Nagarathna,

M.D.M.D., encourage breathing exercises in which I imagined to be too simple while it was bringing prana (vital energy) into my right upper chest. Other therapy included asana, Pranayama, meditation, chanting, lectures on philosophy, and various kriya (internal cleansing practices). I was told to stop practicing Headstand and Shoulderstand in favor of gentle asana coordinated with the breath. In Pune, S.V. Karandikar, a medical doctor, recommended practices with ropes and belts to put the balance on my spine and exercises that taught me to use my shoulder blades to open my upper back.

My experience inspired me to work more over the scientific studies I'd collected in India as well as the West to identify and explain how yoga can both prevent disease and help you recover from it. Here is what I found.

1. Improves Your Flexibility

Yoga helps you to Improves your flexibility; this is one of the first and most obvious benefits of yoga. During your first class, it's possible you won't be able to touch your toes, never mind do a backbend. On the other hand, if you stick with the practices without giving up, you'll notice a gradual loosening, and eventually, poses you thoughts are invisible will become possible. You'll also see that all aches and pains start to disappear. That's no coincidence. Tight hips can strain the knee joint due to improper alignment of the thigh and shinbones. Tight hamstrings can lead to a flattening of the lumbar spine, which can cause back pain.

And inflexibility in muscles and connective tissue, such as fascia and ligaments, can cause poor posture.

2. Builds Muscle Strength

Been strong is a product of hard work, and it does more than look good. This also protects us from conditions like arthritis and back pain, and help prevent falls in older adults. And when you build strength through yoga, you balance it with flexibility. If you just went to the gym and lifted weights, you might develop muscle at the expense of flexibility which is dangerous

3. Perfects Your Posture

Your head is like a bowling ball—big, round, and bulky. When it's balanced directly over an erect spine, it takes much less work for your neck and back muscles to support it. Move it several inches forward, however, and you start to strain those muscles. Hold up that forward-leaning bowling ball for eight or 12 hours a day, and it's no wonder you're tired. And fatigue might not be your only problem. Poor posture can cause back, neck, and other muscle and joint problems. As you slump, your body may compensate by flattening the standard inward curves in your neck and lower back. This can cause pain and degenerative arthritis of the spine.

4. Prevents Cartilage and Joint Breakdown

The practice of yoga enables you to take your joints through their full range of motion. This always helps to avoid decline arthritis or mitigate disability by "Squeezing and soaking" areas of cartilage that typically aren't used.

5. Protects Your Spine

Yoga practices help you preserve your Spinal disks—the shock absorbers between the vertebrae that can herniate and compress nerves—crave movement. If you've got a well-balanced in asana practice with plenty of backbends, forward bends, and twist, you'll be able to maintain your disks flexible.

6. Betters Your Bone Health

Yoga helps to strengthen bones through weight-bearing exercise and helps ward off the risk of early menopause. Many postures in yoga require that you lift your weight some like Downward and upward Facing Dog, it helps strengthen the arm bones, which are particularly vulnerable to osteoporotic fractures. A study which was not published was conducted at California State University, Los Angeles, yoga practice increased bone density in the vertebrae (a small bones which makes up the backbones). Yoga can lower levels of the stress hormone hydrocortisone, which may help keep calcium in the bones.

7. Increases Your Blood Flow

Yoga enables the flowage of your blood in the body system easily. More specifically, the relaxation exercises you learn in yoga will help the circulation of blood, especially in your hands and feet. Yoga also helps in getting more oxygen to your cells, which makes it function better as a result. Twisting poses are thought to twist out venous blood from internal organs and allow oxygenated blood to flow in once the twist is released. Inverted poses, such as Headstand, and Shoulder stand, enable the venous blood from the legs and pelvis to rush back to the heart, where it can be pumped to the lungs to be freshly oxygenated. This always helps in a situation if you have swelling in your legs from heart or kidney problems. Yoga also helps in the boosting level of hemoglobin and red blood cells, which carry oxygen to the tissues. This can play a significant role in the decrease in heart attacks and strokes since blood clots are the primary cause of these killers.

8. Drains Your Lymphs and Boosts Immunity

Yoga helps you to remove your lymph while your freedom is increase. This happened when you contract and stretch muscles, move organs around, and come in and out of yoga postures; with all this, and you increase the drainage of lymph (a viscous fluid rich in immune cells). This helps the lymphatic system fight infection, destroy cancerous cells, and dispose of the toxic waste products of cellular functioning.

9. Ups Your Heart Rate

Yoga practices help you to stabilize your heart rate up. When you regularly get your heart rate into the aerobic range, you lower your risk of heart attack and can relieve depression. It should be noted that not all yoga is aerobic. If you do it forcefully or take flow or Ashtanga classes, it can boost your heart rate into the aerobic range. On the other hand, in a situation when yoga exercises don't get your heart rate up that high can improve cardiovascular conditioning. Studies have shown that yoga practice lowers the resting heart rate, increases endurance, and can improve your maximum uptake of oxygen during exercise—all reflections of enhanced aerobic conditioning.

10. Drops Your Blood Pressure

Yoga helps in the dropping of high blood pressure. If you've got high blood pressure, you might benefit from yoga practices. Two studies of people with hypertension, published in the British medical journal *The Lancet*, compared the effects of Savasana (Corpse Pose) with simply lying on a couch. After three months, Savasana was associated with a 26-point drop in systolic blood pressure (the top number) and a 15-point drop in diastolic blood pressure (the bottom number—and the higher the initial blood pressure, the bigger the fall.

11. Regulates Your Adrenal Glands

Yoga helps to lower cortisol levels. Usually, the adrenal glands secrete cortisol in response to an acute crisis, which temporarily boosts immune function. Peradventure your cortisol levels stay high even after the crisis; they can compromise the immune system. It advisable the cortisol is a boost because temporary boosting of cortisol help with long-term memory, but weak high levels undermine memory and may lead to permanent changes in the brain or permanent defect in the brain.

12. Makes you happier

Feeling sad? Try yoga. It advisable you get up of your feet, rise into a backbend or soar royally into King Dancer Pose. While it's not as simple as that, a study found that a regular yoga practice improved depression and led to a significant increase in serotonin levels and a decrease in the levels of monoamine oxidase (an enzyme that breaks down neurotransmitters) and cortisol. At the University of Wisconsin, Richard Davidson, Ph.D., found that the left prefrontal cortex showed heightened activity in meditators. This finding has been correlated with higher levels of happiness and better immune function. More dramatic left-sided activation was found in dedicated, long-term practitioners.

13. Founds A Healthy Lifestyle

Move more, eat less—that's the proverb of many a dieter. Yoga can help on both fronts. A regular and consistent practice gets you moving, and burns calories and the spiritual and emotional dimensions of your training may encourage you to address any eating and weight problems on a deeper level. Yoga will also inspire you to become a more conscious eater.

14. Lowers Blood Sugar

Yoga lowers blood sugar and LDL (Low-density Lipoprotein) cholesterol and boosts HDL (high-density lipoprotein) cholesterol. People with diabetes, yoga have helped to reduce blood sugar in several ways: it has benefited by lowering cortisol and adrenaline levels. It has also help encouraging weight loss and improving sensitivity to the effects of insulin. Yoga has also contributed to get your blood sugar levels down, and you decrease your risk of diabetic complications, such as blindness, kidney failure, and heart attack.

15. Helps You Focus

An essential component of yoga is focusing on the present, and it helps you to put the past behind and focus on the present. Studies have shown that regular yoga practice improves coordination, reaction time, memory, and even I.Q.I.Q. Scores. It is believed that people who practice Transcendental Meditation demonstrate the ability to solve the crucial problem, they also acquire and recall information better than others probably because they're less distracted by their thoughts or emotions, which can play over and over like an endless tape loop.

16. Relaxes Your System

Yoga encourages and enforces you to relax your mind, slow your breath, and focus on the present, moving the balance from the sympathetic nervous system (or the fight-or-flight response) to the parasympathetic nervous system. Yoga decreases blood pressure and increases blood flow to the intestines and reproductive organs—comprising what Herbert Benson, M.D.M.D., calls the relaxation response. It also lowers breathing and heart rates, which improve the maximum uptake of oxygen during exercise.

17. Improves Your Balance

Regularly practicing yoga increases the ability to feel what your body is doing and where it is in space and improves balance. People with bad posture or incorrect movement patterns will always have poor proprioception, which has been linked to knee problems and back pains. This resulted in the increment of older adults into independence and delayed admission to a nursing home or never entering one at all. For the young once, postures like Tree Pose can make us feel less rickety on and off the mat.

18. Maintains Your Nervous System

Some advanced yoga practices can control our bodies in extraordinary ways, and yoga is said to keep our nervous system, many of which are mediated by the nervous system. Scientists have monitored yogis who could bring unusual heart rhythms which generate specific brain-wave patterns, and, using a meditation formant, raise the temperature of their hands by 15 degrees Fahrenheit. If it is possible to do that, using yoga practices. Yoga could teach you how to improve blood flow to your pelvis if you're trying to get pregnant or brings relaxation when you're having trouble falling asleep.

19. Releases Tension In Your Limbs

Do you ever notice yourself holding the telephone or a steering wheel with a death grip or scrunching your face when staring at a computer screen? Tensions in your limbs cause these. These unconscious habits can lead to muscle fatigue and soreness in the wrists, arms, shoulders, neck, and face, which can increase stress and worsen your mood (Mood swing).

As you begin the practice yoga, you begin to realize where you hold tension: It might be in your tongue, your eyes, or the muscles of your face and neck. If you simply tune in, you may be able to release some tension in the tongue and eyes. With bigger muscles like the quadriceps, trapezius, and buttocks, it may take years of practice to learn how to relax them.

20. Helps You Sleep Deeper

Stimulation is functional, but too much of it creates a problem for the nervous system. Yoga can provide relief from the hustle and bustle of modern life and gives you a dip sleep after all tensions and stress have been release.

21. Boosts Your Immune System Functionality

Yoga (Asana and Pranayama) probably improve immune function, but research has shown that meditation has the most reliable scientific support in promoting the immune system. It appears to have a beneficial effect on the functioning of the immune system, boosting it when needed (for example, raising antibody levels in response to a vaccine) and lowering it when needed (for instance, mitigating an inappropriately aggressive immune function in an autoimmune disease like psoriasis).

22. Gives Your Lungs Room To Breathe

Yoga practices enable you to take fewer breaths of higher volume. A study published in The Lancet during the year 1998 taught a yogic technique known as "Complete Breathing" to people with lung problems due to mass heart failure. After one month, their average respiratory rate decreased from 13.4 breaths per minute to 7.6, which was a great recovering. Meanwhile, their exercise throughput increased significantly, as did the oxygen saturation of their blood. Also, yoga has been shown to improve various measures of lung function, including the maximum volume of the breath and the efficiency of the respiration.

Yoga also promotes breathing through the nose, which filters the air, warms it (cold, dry air is more likely to trigger an asthma attack in sensitive people), and humidifies it, removing pollen and dirt and other things you'd instead not take into your lungs.

23. Prevents I.B.S. and Other Digestive Problems

Ulcers, irritable bowel syndrome, constipation; these entire can be exacerbated by stress. So if you stress less, you'll suffer less. Yoga can ease constipation, and theoretically, it lowers the risk of colon cancer.

24. Gives You Peace of Mind

Yoga subdues the fluctuations of the brain, according to Patanjali's Yoga Sutra. In other words, it slows down the mental loops of frustration, regret, anger, fear, and desire that can cause stress. Since stress is implicated in so many health problems—from migraines and insomnia to lupus, M.S.M.S., eczema, high blood pressure, and heart attacks—if you learn to quiet your mind, you'll be likely to live longer and healthier.

25. Increases Your Self-esteem

Many of us suffer from chronic low self-esteem. If you handle this negatively, take drugs, overeat, work too hard, sleep around, you may pay the price in poorer health physically, mentally, and spiritually. If you take a positive approach and practice yoga, you'll sense, initially in brief glimpses and later in more sustained views, that you're worthwhile or, as yogic philosophy teaches, that you are a manifestation of the Divine. If you practice regularly with the intention of self-examination and betterment, not just as a substitute for an aerobics class, you can access a different side of yourself. You'll experience feelings of gratitude, empathy, and forgiveness as well as a sense that you're part of something bigger. While better health is not the goal of spirituality, it's often a by-product, as documented by repeated scientific studies.

26. Eases Your Pain

Yoga can ease your pain. According to several studies of asana, meditation or combination of the two reduced pain in people with arthritis, back pain, fibromyalgia, carpal tunnel syndrome, and other chronic conditions. When you relieve your pain, your mood improves, you're more inclined to be active, and you don't need as much medication.

27. Gives You Inner Strength

Yoga can help you make changes in your life. It does not change you, but it helps to change how you interact with the experience. That might be its greatest strength. Tapa, the Sanskrit word for "Heat," is the fire, the discipline that fuels yoga practice and that regular exercise builds. The tapas you develop can be extended to the rest of your life to overcome inertia and change dysfunctional habits. You may find that without making a particular effort to change things, you start to eat better, exercise more, or finally quit smoking after years of failed attempts.

28. Connects You With Guidance

Good yoga teachers can do wonders for your health. Exceptional ones do more than guide you through the postures. They can adjust your position, gauge when you should go more in-depth in poses or back off, deliver hard truths with compassion, help you relax, and enhance and personalize your practice. A respectful relationship with a teacher goes a long way toward promoting your health.

29. Help Keep You Drug-free

If your medicine cabinet looks like a pharmacy, maybe it's time to try yoga. Studies show that people with asthma, high blood pressure, Type II diabetes (formerly called adult-onset diabetes), and obsessive-compulsive disorder have shown that yoga helped them lower their dosage of medications and sometimes get off them entirely. You'll spend less money on drugs, and you're less likely to suffer side effects and risk dangerous drug interactions.

30. Builds Awareness For Transformation

Yoga and meditation build awareness. And the more aware you are, the easier it is to break free of destructive emotions like anger. Studies suggest that chronic anger and hostility are as strongly linked to heart attacks as are smoking, diabetes, and elevated cholesterol. Yoga appears to reduce violence by increasing feelings of compassion and interconnection and by calming the nervous system and the mind. It also increases your ability to step back from the drama of your own life, to remain steady in the face of bad news or unsettling events. You can still react quickly when you need to—and there's evidence that yoga speeds reaction time—but you can take that split second to choose a more thoughtful approach, reducing suffering for yourself and others.

31. **Benefits Your Relationships**

Love may not conquer all, but it certainly can aid in healing. Cultivating the emotional support of friends, family, and community has been demonstrated repeatedly to improve health and healing. Regular yoga practice helps develop friendliness, compassion, and greater equanimity. Along with yogic philosophy's emphasis on avoiding harm to others, telling the truth, and taking only what you need, this may improve many of your relationships.

32. **Guides Your Body's Healing In Your Mind's Eye**

If you contemplate an image in your mind's eye, as you do in yoga Nidra and other practices, you can effect change in your body. Several studies have found that guided imagery reduced postoperative pain, decreased the frequency of headaches, and improved the quality of life for people with cancer and H.I.V.

33. **Helps You Serve Others**

Karma yoga (service to others) is integral to yogic philosophy. And while you may not be inclined to serve others, your health might improve if you do. A study at the University of Michigan found that older people who volunteered a little less than an hour per week were three times as likely to be alive seven years later. Serving others can give meaning to your life, and your problems may not seem so daunting when you see what other people are dealing with.

34. Supports Your Connective Tissue

Yoga helps to improve your health; you might probably notice a lot of overlap, that's because they're intensely interwoven. Change your posture, and you change the way you breathe. This is one of the great lessons of yoga: Everything is connected—your hipbone to your anklebone, you to your community, your community to the world. This interconnection is vital to understanding yoga. This holistic system simultaneously taps into many mechanisms that have additive and even multiplicative effects. This synergy may be the most important way of all that yoga heals.

Chapter 4 - Yoga For Everyone

Yoga practitioners have proved that yoga is for everyone, therefore, it's time to roll out our yoga mat and discover the combination and usefulness of physical and mental exercises that, for thousands of years, the yoga practices have been hooked around the globe. The beauty of yoga is that you don't have to be a yogi or yogini to reap the benefits. Whether you are young or old, overweight, or fit, yoga has way calmed the mind and strengthens the body. Don't be intimidated by yoga vocabularies, lingo, fancy yoga studios, and complicated poses. Yoga is for everyone, and everyone can participate in yoga training.

10 Yoga Poses You Need To Know

The building blocks of yoga are poses. These are good ones to learn as you build a regular yoga practice.

These ten poses are a complete yoga workout, i.e., there are the basics of yoga.

Move slowly through each pose, remembering to breathe as you move. Pause after any pose you find difficult, especially if you are short of breath, and start again when your breathing returns to normal. The idea is to hold each pose for a few, slow breaths before moving on to the next one.

Child's Pose

This calming pose is a good default pause position. This pose can also be used to rest and relax before continuing to your next posture. It politely stretches your lower back, thighs, hips, knees, and ankles and relaxes your spine, shoulders, and neck.

Do it: When you want to get a beautiful, gentle stretch through your neck spine and hips.

Skip it: If you have knee injuries or ankle problems, please avoid this pose. Avoid also, if you have high blood pressure or are pregnant.

Modify: You can launch this pose by resting your head or support it on a cushion or block. You can place a rolled towel under your ankles if they are uncomfortable.

Be mindful: Focus on relaxing the muscles of the spine and lower back as you breathe.

This should be the pose you should usually do whenever you need to rest for a moment during a yoga workout.

Downward-Facing Dog

This helps in strengthens the arms, shoulders, and back while stretching the hamstrings, calves, and arches of your feet. It can also be called a back pain reliever

Do it: To help relieve back pain.

Skip it: This kind pose is not advisable for people that have carpal tunnel syndrome or other wrist problems; people with have high blood pressure or are in the late stages of pregnancy.

Modify: This kind of pose can be lunched with your elbows on the ground, which automatically takes the weight off your wrists. You can also use blocks under your hands, which may feel more comfortable.

Be mindful: you should focus on distributing the weight evenly through your palms while lifting your hips up and down, away from your shoulders.

Plank Pose

This is a frequent exercise that can be practiced by everyone, and plank enables you to build strength in the core, shoulders, arms, and legs.

Do it: Plank pose is right for you if you are looking to tone your abs and build strength in your upper body.

Skip it: Stay away from plank pose if you suffer from carpal tunnel syndrome. You might also skip or modify it if you have low back pain. It can be hard on your wrist.

Modify: You can modify it by placing your knees on the floor.

Be Mindful: As you do a plank, imagine the back of your neck and spine lengthening.

This standard pose can build strength in the core, shoulders, arms, and legs.

Four-Limbed Staff Pose

It's normal after the plank posture the push-up variation (four-limbed staff pose) follow in a standard yoga sequence. This pose helps you to determine if you want to eventually work on more advanced poses such as arm balances or inversions.

Do it: Like plank, this pose helps in strengthens the arms and wrists and tones the abdomen.

Skip it: If you have carpal tunnel syndrome, lower back pain, a shoulder injury, or you are pregnant.

Modify: It's a good idea for beginners to modify the pose by keeping your knees on the floor.

Be Mindful: Press your palms evenly into the floor and lift your shoulders away from the floor as you hold this pose.

This pose builds strength in the arms, shoulders, wrists, and back and helps tone the abdomen.

Cobra Pose

This is a back-bending pose that helps in strengthening the back muscles, increase spinal flexibility, and stretches the chest, shoulders, and abdomen.

Do it: This post is suitable for strengthening the back muscles.

Skip it: Avoid if you have arthritis in your spine or neck, a low-back injury or carpal tunnel syndrome.

Modify: Just lift a few inches, and don't attempt to straighten your arms.

Be mindful: Try to keep your umbilicus drawing up away from the floor as you hold this pose.

Tree Pose

This is a significant pose for balance improvement, beyond helping to improve your balance; it can also strengthen your core, ankles, calves, thighs, and spine.

Do it: This is great for working on your balance and posture.

Skip it: You may decide to skip this pose if you have low blood pressure or any medical conditions that affect your balance,

Modify: Place one of your hands on a wall for support.

Be mindful: Focus on your breath in and out as you hold this pose.

This balancing pose (tree pose) is one of the most recognized poses in modern yoga.

Triangle Pose

Triangle pose, this is one part of many yoga sequences that helps to build strength in the legs and stretches the hips, hamstrings chest, shoulders, groins, spine, and calves. It can also help increase mobility in the hips and neck.

Do it: This pose is excellent once you decide to build strength and endurance.

Skip it: It advisable you avoid this pose if you have a headache or low blood pressure.

Modify: If you have high blood pressure, turn your head to gaze downward in the final pose. If you have neck problems, don't turn your head to look upward; look straight ahead and keep both sides of the neck long.

Be mindful: Keep lifting your raised arm toward the ceiling. It helps keep the pose buoyant.

This is a particular pose and which can be found in many yoga sequences.

Seated Half-Spinal Twist Pose

This is a pose that can help relieve tension in the middle of your back. It's a twisting pose that can increase the flexibility in your back while stretching the shoulders, hips, and chest.

Do it: To release tight muscles around the shoulders and upper and lower back.

Skip it: If you have a back injury.

Modify: If bending your right knee is uncomfortable or unsuitable for you to do, keep it straight out in front of you.

Be Mindful: Lift your trunk with each inhale, and twist as you exhale.

Want to relieve the tension in your back?

Bridge Pose

This is also being called a back-bending pose, which enables you to stretches the muscles of the chest, back, and neck. It also builds strength in the back and hamstring muscles.

Do it: This pose will help you open your upper chest, especially those who sit all day.

Skip it: Avoid this pose if you have a neck injury.

Modify: Place a block between your thighs to enable your legs and feet in proper alignment. Or you can place a block under your pelvis if your lower back is paining you.

Be Mindful: While holding this pose, try to keep your chest lifted and your sternum toward your chin.

Bridge pose is from the back-bending family of yoga poses, which is excellent for stretching the muscles of the chest.

Corpse Pose

Corpse pose allows for a moment of relaxation, but some people find it challenging to stay still in this pose for an extended period. However, the more you try this pose, the easier it is to sink into a relaxing. Just like the reality of life, yoga classes typically end with this pose.

Do it: Always!

Skip it: If you don't want to have a moment's peace.

Modify: Place a blanket under your head, if that feels more comfortable. If the lower back is bothering you, you can roll up a rug and place that under your knees.

Be Mindful: Feel the weight of your body sinking into your mat one part at a time.

Chapter 5 - Yoga And Meditation

Before yoga was a popular physical exercise, it was mainly a meditation practice for thousands of years,

Mindfulness With Yoga

During the process of learning yoga poses, you will be guild on how to notice your breath and the way your body moves during the exercises. This is the primary foundation of a mind-body connection. A complete series of yoga exercises allows you to scan your entire body, noting the way you feel as you move through the poses. You may begin to realize that one side of your body feels different than the other during a stretch, or that it's easier to balance on your right leg over your left leg, or that certain poses help ease tension in your neck.

With these applications, yoga turns into physical exercise tools that help students become more mindful and even learn to meditate.

Stephen Cope, who teaches yoga and mindfulness at Kripalu Center for Yoga and Health in Massachusetts, has written that learning to focus through yoga poses can help us outside of yoga class.

It helps you in learning to be aware of your posture at your desk, or when you walk, for example, this can be the first step to make improvements that will make you move more quickly and feel better all the time.

The Breath

This can be a crucial part of yoga; not only do they help you to stay focused while practicing yoga, but they can also help reduce stress and relax the nervous system and calm the mind.

Yoga breathing techniques also offer a way into meditation, says Elena Brower, a yoga and meditation teacher and the author of "Art of Attention." Ms. Brower says that more people who have in recent years focused on the physical aspects of yoga are moving toward meditation, as they find "They have an increasing need to have time to reflect, release, and recalibrate."

Here are a few types of breathing techniques that may be included in a yoga class:

Abdominal Breathing: Also called belly breathing, it is the most common breathing technique you'll find in basic yoga. It helps aid healthy and efficient breathing in general.

Inflate your abdomen as you inhale.

Victorious Breath: This enables you to slow and smooth the flow of breath. It is often used in flow classes to help students control their breathing as they move through the poses.

Constrict the muscles in the back of your throat and breathe in and out with your mouth closed.

Make sure the sound should be audible to you only; your neighbor doesn't necessarily need to hear it. Some say this sounds like Darth Vader; others say it seems like the ocean.

Interval or Interrupted Breathing: In this kind of breathing, the students are instructed to pauses and hold the breath during the inhalation and exhalation. It is an excellent way to begin to learn to control the breath, especially if you are looking to try more advanced yoga breathing techniques.

Try it:

- Inhale fully.
- Release one-third of the breath
- Pause
- Release another third of the breath
- Pause
- Exhale the rest of the breath
- Repeat

If you like, you can then do a couple of rounds of interrupted breathing during exhalation.

Alternate nostril breathing: This technique helps in balancing the nervous system and is a good idea to try before meditation

Try it:

- Hold one nostril closed and inhale through the open nose
- Exhale through the open nostril
- Switch your hands and block the open nostril, releasing the closed nose
- Inhale through the open nostril and exhale
- Repeat several times

You don't need anything to start a yoga practice, but here's what you may want as you progress.

Yoga Mats

Almost all yoga studios and gyms center offer mats, but it advisable you buy a mat for hygiene and because mats differ in material, density and stickiness. You may find you develop a strong preference for a specific type of mat.

Choose a mat that prevents you from slipping and sliding, as that will give you a stable base for changing from one pose to the next. Ensure your mat is clean regularly with antibacterial wipes. If you have the intention to rent mats at the studio or gym, it would be a good idea to carry around a small packet of antibacterial wipes to clean your rental mat for your safety.

Clothes

Any comfortable clothing is recommended. Workout clothes would generally work well for a yoga class. However, avoid clothes that are too loose-fitting because it may get in the way if you progress into headstand and handstand poses.

Beginning a Yoga Practice

If you desire to achieve the full benefits of yoga, it's essential to make it a way of life that is finding a way to make it a regular part of your routine.

Creating a Habit

The most important thing to remember when starting a yoga practice (or any new health habit) is that the key to success is doing it routinely. Without regular exercise, the goal may not be achieved. Start small and manageable, says Dr. McCall. Ten or 15 minutes a day of yoga may be more valuable than going to one class a week. "I would rather have a student succeed at doing a one-minute-a-day practice than fail at doing a five-minute-a-day practice," says Dr. McCall.

Hopefully, as you begin to see the benefits of your daily practice, however short, chances are you will be convinced to do more.

Find a Class

Yoga can be done at home, but for a beginner, it is advisable to try a class or get an instructor in a private or group setting to be sure you are doing the yoga exercises correctly and safely. If you have any specific medical concerns, check with a doctor before beginning to see what types of yoga might be best for you.

Look for an experienced yoga instructor who has at least a 200-hour teaching certificate from a teacher-training program accredited with the Yoga Alliance. Those programs include training on injury prevention

Look for yoga studios or gyms that provide good slip-resistant mats (if you are planning on renting a mat) and sturdy, clean blocks for support. If you do rent a mat, make sure there is antibacterial spray or cloths available for you to wipe down your mat before and after use.

What Class is Right for Me?

It is essential to know the best class that fits your personality. There are many styles of yoga classes taught today. Some are very physically challenging and will leave you sweating; others are gentle and restorative. Some teachers play music in class; others don't. Some categories include references to yoga philosophy and spirituality; others don't.

Here are a few types of classes your yoga studio or gym may offer:

Hatha: This is the most yoga styles being taught in America. Hatha yoga is generally referred to as the physical part of yoga, rather than yoga philosophy or meditation. A Hatha yoga class is likely to be a combination of poses and breathing exercises, but it's hard to know whether it will be challenging or gentle. Check with the school or the teacher to find more about the level of classes that are described only as Hatha yoga.

Ashtanga Yoga: Some students think that yoga is not a workout; this is because they haven't tried an Ashtanga class. Ashtanga yoga is a challenging style of yoga that is centered on a progressive series of yoga sequences. The categories include advanced poses, such as arm balances and inversions, including headstands and shoulder stands. Some students practice on their own under the guidance of a teacher, but beginner students are strongly advised to study with an experienced teacher. Ashtanga classes will also often include teachings in yoga philosophy.

Power Yoga: Power yoga is a challenging style of yoga, which aims at strength-building just as its name suggests, These classes will include advanced poses and inversions like headstands and handstands that require a lot of strength.

Vinyasa or Flow: These classes consist of an energetic flowing sequence of yoga poses, which includes depending on the level of advanced poses, such as arm balances, headstands, shoulder stands, and handstands. Vinyasa classes always deal with the musical accompaniment of the teacher's choosing.

Iyengar: Iyengar teaches you how your muscles and joints work together. Iyengar yoga focuses on the precision of your yoga poses. Iyengar classes use items including blankets, blocks, straps, and bolsters, to help students do poses that they wouldn't be able to do otherwise

Bikram or Hot Yoga: Do you like the heat? Do you like everywhere to be warm?

Bikram yoga is what you need. Bikram yoga has a set of 26 poses series performed in a room heated to 105 degrees, which is said to allow for deeper stretching and provide for a better cardiovascular workout. Bikram classes are always done in places with mirrors. Bikram yoga is referred to as any yoga class that is done in a heated room — generally from 80 to 110 degrees.

Restorative Yoga: This yoga gives you more relaxation pose if you are looking for a little more relaxation from your yoga class, restorative yoga is for you. This yoga style usually involves a few restful poses that are held for long periods. Restorative poses include light twists, seated forward folds, and gentle backbends, traditionally done with the assistance of many props, including blankets, blocks, and bolsters.

Yin Yoga: Looking for a new kind of stretching experience? Yin yoga is aimed at stretching the connective tissue around the pelvis, sacrum, spine, and knees to promote flexibility. Poses are held for a more extended amount of time in yin yoga classes, generally from three to five minutes. It is a quiet style of yoga, and will quickly show you how good you are at sitting still.

Class Etiquette

Yoga students are expected to turn your cellphone off before class and expected to be in class on time students must learn to respect their instructor and be respectful of one another. Crowded classes can mean that students will be aligned mat-to-mat, so they may not have a lot of room around you for personal belongings. Most yoga classrooms have shelves for your valuables, drinks, and other personal items.

For Bikram or hot yoga classes, bring a towel. You are going to sweat, and it will help prevent slipping.

Classes usually begin with a brief introduction by the teacher or instructor that may include a focus or theme for the day, such as backbends or particular poses. Then the teacher often will instruct the class to chant the word "Om" together. (Om is a Sanskrit term that connotes the connectivity of all things in the universe.)

To "Om" or not to "Om"? There is no obligation to chant, but you should at least remain quiet during that time.

Some breathing techniques taught in yoga classes are meant to be loud, and others are not. Students should take cues from the teacher.

If there is a need for you to leave early, try to tell the teacher ahead of time, and, if you can't, position yourself near the back of the room to avoid distraction.

A note to the over-achiever: Trying too hard often leads to injury. Being aware of your physical limitations and when you need to modify a pose will be more beneficial to your body than reaching to be the most flexible or most reliable in the class.

Chapter 6 - Why Is Breathing So Important In Yoga?

Why is there so much focus on the breath in yoga? What is the relationship between yoga and breath, and why is it so important (besides the fact that it keeps us alive)?

In a typical yoga class, we are instructed to connect to our breath, consciously breathe, breathe deeply, and retain our breath. What impact does the breath have on us, what benefit does breath have on us apart from the fact that it keeps us alive, what impact does it have on our yoga practice?

1. Breath and Length of Life
2. Conscious Breathing

It is said that if you breathe 15 times per minute, you will live to 75 or 80 years. If you breathe ten times per minute, you will live to 100. The speed at which you breathe will dictate the length of life. If you breathe fast, your life will be shortened. This is why dogs have short lives.

We are instructed to "Breathe Consciously" when we are in yoga class. Breathing consciously is a way of life in yoga, and it assists us in connecting with the subtle energy within. It is through the breath that we can navigate different levels of consciousness. Moreover, breathing consciously has a biological effect on our mental, emotional, and physical state.

Firstly, connecting with your breath is a method for being present. When you concentrate on each aspect of the breathing process, you automatically let go of the past and future, and you are focused on the moment inside the breath. This is why breathing consciously is a meditation on its own, but this is just the beginning of why conscious breathing is important.

When you breathe consciously, you activate a different part of your brain. Unconscious breathing is controlled by the medulla oblongata in the brain stem, the primitive part of the brain, while conscious breathing comes from the more evolved areas of the brain in the cerebral cortex. So conscious breathing stimulates the cerebral cortex and the more evolved areas of the brain. Consciously breathing sends impulses from the cortex to the connecting areas that impact emotions. Activating the cerebral cortex has a relaxing and balancing effect on the emotions. In essence, by consciously breathing, you are controlling which aspects of the mind dominate, causing your consciousness to rise from the primitive/instinctual to the evolved/elevated.

Controlling the Breath

Changing the breathing pattern makes you produce different states of mind. Slowing down the breath has an impact on your emotional state. The cerebral cortex is activated through consciously slowing down the release of breath. Then the cerebral cortex sends inhibitory impulses to the respiratory center in the midbrain. These inhibitory impulses from the cortex overflow into the area of the hypothalamus, which is concerned with emotions, and relax this area. This is why slowing down the breath has a soothing effect on your emotional state.

Channels of Subtle Energy

Do you know that breath controls the body, mind, and emotions? There are 72,000 channels where the subtle energy flows throughout the body. There are three most important nadis (channels), namely: Ida, Pingala, and Sushumna.

The Ida Nadi begins at the Muladhara Chakra, courses through the chakras and ends in the left nostril. Ida is aligned with the moon energy and has a calming and cooling effect.

The Pingala Nadi originates at the Muladhara Chakra, courses through the chakras and ends in the right nostril. It is associated with solar energy and has a heating effect.

The Sushumna Nadi is the central channel. This is the Nadi that the Kundalini energy travels. It is associated with balance.

During the day, the left and right nostrils alternate in which one dominates. This is accomplished through erectile tissue in the nasal passage that inflates with blood to cut off or reduce the flow of air. One of the nostrils will dominate based on your mental, emotional, and physical state. They alternate throughout the day. As they change over, the Sushumna is activated, but only for a couple of minutes. The key is to activate Sushumna for a longer period. This is accomplished when both the Ida and Pingala are flowing evenly.

Prana and Pranayama

The yoga we teach us how to control prana, the vital force, through Pranayama. We use the breath in Pranayama to learn to control prana, but don't confuse prana with the breath. Prana is the energy that actives the lungs. It does not actives the breath. The breath method is the easiest method for training prana. Once you are able to control prana through Pranayama, you are better able to control the movement of prana to other organs and areas of the body.

The breath being the mode of Pranayama, we focus on the three stages of respiration: inhalation (pooka), retention (kumbhaka), and exhalation (rechaka). However, according to yogic texts, Pranayama is retention. Inhalation and exhalation are methods for affecting retention.

Kumbhaka or retention of the breath has a physiological effect on the brain. First, it provides more opportunities for the cells to absorb oxygen and eliminate more carbon dioxide. This has a calming effect on the mental and emotional body. In fact, scientific studies have proven that slight increases in carbon dioxide for a short amount of time reduce anxiety levels. However, it is only beneficial up to a certain level. Carbon dioxide becomes very harmful, even fatal at high levels.

Furthermore, when the breath is retained, the brain panics because the carbon dioxide levels increase. Increased carbon dioxide levels stimulate the brain's capillaries to dilate. In this way, more capillaries in the brain are opened up to improve cerebral circulation. This builds up an immense amount of nervous energy in the brain, forcing the creation of new neural pathways and the activation of dormant centers; the brain is activated and awakened!

Breath and Sound

Every vibration has sound. Breath is a vibration; it also has sound. The Yoga Chudamani Upanishads states at a particular level of consciousness the breath has a sound it gives. According to the Upanishads, the sound of the breath is *"So"* during inhalation and *"Ham"* during exhalation.

When you withdraw your senses from the external and switch to the internal, then you can hear the sound of the breath. By mentally chanting (So and ham), the mantra manifests as an audible sound in the inner ear. In Kundalini Yoga, we mentally chant *Sat* on the inhale and *Nam* on the exhale, which serves the same purpose.

Mind, Prana, and Breath

Let assumes that the breath is like the oil in a car, prana as the gasoline, and the mind as the engine. By understanding the relationship between these three, you are better equipped to navigate your life to a higher elevation and repair it when it breaks down. The yoga mat is just the starting point of your journey.

Best Yoga Breathing Exercises

In yoga, we call the branch dedicated to our breathing techniques, Pranayama, which means breath control.

Breathing exercises are a very useful tool in our daily lives; they are a huge part of any yoga practice,

Before you get started, it's always important to try to take a few relaxed breaths before and after each exercise. Start with just 30 seconds per exercise, and this helps in building a long increment of time as your body is ready. If you get dizzy, simply stop and relax for a few minutes,

There is a group of different techniques you can try utilizing for different effects. Here are just a few in no particular order.

1. Lion's Breath

This breath control activity encourages a sudden release and invites a little playfulness into the practice. This is one of the most fun breathing practices, especially for kids. It is also a great addition to an adult class on Friday evenings or

Saturday mornings, when everyone is ready to let go of the week they have had, and embrace the weekend.

Lion's breath involves inhaling deeply through your nose, then leaning your head back and opening your mouth very wide to exhale loudly while sticking your tongue out. Try practicing this while raising your arms up on the inhale and forming cactus arms with your exhale to accentuate the relieving effects.

2. **Breath of Fire**

This breath is used in Bikram classes; this practice is very warming as the name itself implies. It is great for warming up the abdominal muscles and ignites Tapas, or heat, in the organs. This is superb for a practice that is focused on detoxing.

Practice Breath of Fire by sitting tall, inhaling gently through your nose, then vigorously pumping you exhale out through your nose while pulling your navel in repeatedly and in short spurts. Each pulls in with your belly exerts another exhale quickly after the last. Make your inhales and exhales even in force, depth, and time.

3. **Skull Cleanser**

This is also known as Kapalabhati Breathing, and this technique helps in raising your energy level dramatically. It is another cleansing breath exercise. Basically, it is the same as the Breath of Fire technique, but with a larger emphasis on the exhale, and with your arms straight up above your head to promote lymph circulation through the upper body.

Hold your hands in the mudra of your choice. For example, try Apana Mudra for invoking the future. Simply make your hands look like a dog's head with the ring and middle finger resting on your thumb in a triangle, stick your pinkie and pointer finger straight up like ears.

4. Three-Part Breathing

This method works slowly, smoothly, and process in a super relaxing way and is wonderful for insomnia, anxiety, stress, and frustrating situations. The three Part Breathing calms the mind and soothes the muscles. It is an amazing way to end a late evening practice or begin a restorative practice.

It begins by placing one hand on your upper chest and the other on your navel. Inhale into your chest, then your upper abdomen, and finally puff your belly out like a balloon. Slowly release the breath in the same way, smoothly exhaling the air from your belly, then your upper abdomen, then your chest.

5. Alternate Nostril Breathing

This breathing exercise takes focus and clarity to prevent getting perplexed and to remember where you are in the process. For this reason, it is best used before an exam or when you are trying to ignite focus and discipline for any reason. This method helps in calming down as it clears the mind while focusing; so many people will use it before bed if they tend to overthink stuff at night.

Practice this technique by placing your right middle and pointer fingers in the palm of your hand, leaving just your pinkie and ring fingers and your thumb free. Take your right thumb over your right nostril and inhale through the left nostril. Now take your ring finger and place it over your left nostril to exhale through the right nostril.

Next, leave your hand as it is and inhale through the left nostril, then switch, placing your thumb over your right nostril and exhaling through the left nostril. Repeat this until you are finished with your breathing exercise.

The first few times you try this one, you may get your left and right confused. Don't give up; you're not alone in that struggle. Try to remember that each time you inhale, you are sealing the breath in and that is when you switch sides.

6. Bellows Breath

Bellows Breath is very, very invigorating and is a wonderful way to begin an early morning Power yoga practice or to wake yourself up in the middle of a meeting or long lecture.

Raise your hands up to the sky in little fists, while the fingers splayed out wide. Inhale through your mouth, and with every exhale, drop your elbows into your side body and make a "HA" sound from the bottom of your diaphragm.

Don't be afraid to be loud here, as this is incredibly freeing and releases any pent up energy, stagnation, or frustrations very quickly.

7. Ujjayi Breath

This technique is useful for calming the mind and the nervous system in difficult situations both on and off the mat. It is the most used breathing technique. It is always easy to perform during any physical practice. It sounds like the ocean and can cool you off very quickly.

Practice Ujjayi breathing by inhaling and exhaling through your nose. Drag the breath along the back of your throat so that it creates a gentle hissing sound and feels like sipping a cool drink through a straw. Try to make each inhale last as long as the exhale and take each breathe a little deeper than the last until your breathing is long and smooth.

Practice your breathing techniques as often as possible. Being able to control your breath will deepen your physical practice dramatically, and will help you take each posture longer, deeper, and more healthfully.

Beyond that, it will change your emotional health and allow you to stay cool as a cucumber in arduous situations down the line.

Chapter 7 - Yoga Meditation

What is meditation? And how and why would I do it? Get the answers. It should be noted that you don't need to formally meditate to practice hatha yoga nor is the practice of hatha yoga compulsory to meditate; these two practices support each another. Nevertheless in your practice of yoga, you've improved both your abilities to concentrate and to relax the two most important requirements for a meditation practice. Now you can deepen your understanding of what meditation is and begin a practice of your own.

What Is Meditation?

Meditation is about training in awareness and getting a healthy sense of perspective. It is not about becoming a new person or even a better person.

An exquisite methodology exists within the yoga tradition that is designed to reveal the coming interconnectedness of every living thing. This fundamental unity is referred to as *Advaita*. Meditation is the actual experience of this union.

In the Yoga Sutra, Patanjali gives instructions on how to meditate and portray what factors constitute a meditation practice. The second sutra in the first chapter states that yoga (or union) happens when the mind becomes quiet. This mental calmness is created by bringing the body, mind, and senses into balance which, in turn, relaxes the nervous system. Patanjali goes on to explain that meditation begins when we notice that our never-ending pursuit to possess things and our succession craving for pleasure and security can never be satisfied. When we finally realize this, our external pursuit turns inward, and we have shifted into the realm of meditation.

By dictionary definition, "Meditation" means to reflect upon, ponder, or contemplate. It can also denote a devotional exercise of contemplation or a contemplative discourse of a religious or philosophical nature. The word meditate comes from the Latin *meditari*, which means to think about or consider. *Med* is the root of this word and means "To take appropriate measures." In our culture, to meditate can be interpreted in several ways. For instance, you might meditate on or consider a course of action regarding your child's education, or a career change that would entail a move across the country. Viewing a powerful movie or play, you may be moved to meditate upon—or ponder—the moral issues plaguing today's society.

In the yogic context, meditation, or *dhyana*, is defined more specifically as a state of pure consciousness. It is the seventh stage, or limb, of the yogic path and follows *Dharana*, the art of concentration. Dhyana, in turn, precedes *samadhi,* the state of final freedom or enlightenment, the last step in Patanjali's eight-limbed system. These three limbs—Dharana (concentration), Dhyana (meditation), and Samadhi (ecstasy)—are inextricably linked and collectively referred to as *samyama,* the inner practice, or subtle discipline, of the yogic path.

Recall that the first four limbs— *Yama* (ethics), N*iyama* (self-discipline), *Asana* (posture), and *Pranayama* (life-force extension)—are considered external disciplines. In the fifth step, pratyahara represents the withdrawal of the senses. This physical withdrawal arises out of the practice of the first four steps and links the external to the internal. When we are grounded physically and mentally we are sharply aware of our senses yet disengaged at the same time. Without this ability to remain isolated yet observant, it is not possible to meditate. Even though you need to be able to concentrate in order to meditate, meditation is more than concentration. It ultimately evolves into an expanded state of awareness.

When we concentrate, we direct our minds toward what appears to be an object apart from ourselves. We become acquainted with this object and establish contact with it. To shift into the meditation realm, however, we need to become involved with this object; we need to communicate with it. The result of this exchange, of course, is a deep awareness that there is no difference between us (as the subject) and that which we concentrate or meditate upon (the object). This brings us to the state of samadhi, or self-realization.

A good way to understand this is to think about the development of a relationship. First, we meet someone and then by spending time together, listening to, and sharing with each other, we develop a relationship. In the next stage, we blend with this person in the form of a deep friendship, partnership, or marriage. The "You" and "Me" become "Us."

According to the Yoga Sutra, our pain and suffering are created by the misperception that we are separate from nature. The realization that we aren't separate may be experienced casual without effort. However, most of us need guidance. Patanjali's eight-limbed system provides us with the framework we need.

5 Different Ways to Meditate

Just as there are numerous styles of hatha yoga, so there are many ways to meditate. The first stage of meditation is to concentrate on a specific object. With the eyes either opened or closed. Silently repeating a word or phrase, audibly reciting a prayer or chant, visualizing an image, such as a deity, or focusing on an object such as a lighted candle in front of you are all commonly recommended points of focus. Observing or counting your breaths and noticing bodily sensations are also optional focal points. Let's take a closer look at the 5 way to meditate

The Use of Sound

This method is always been employed by Mantra yoga, it could sound, phrase, or affirmation as a point of focus. The word mantra comes from *man*, which means "To Think," and *tra*, which suggests "Instrumentality." Therefore, the mantra is an instrument of thought. It also has come to mean "Protecting the person who receives it." Traditionally, you can only receive a mantra from a teacher, one who knows you and your particular needs. The act of repeating your mantra is called *Japa*, which means recitation. Just as meditative prayer and affirmation need to be stated with purpose and feeling, a mantra meditation practice requires conscious engagement on the part of the mediator. Maharishi Mahesh Yogi's Transcendental Meditation (TM) espouses the practice of mantra yoga.

Chanting, an extension of mantra yoga is a powerful way to enter into meditation. Longer than a mantra, a chant involves both rhythm and pitch. Western traditions use chants and hymns to invoke the name of God, to inspire, and to produce a spiritual awakening. During the Vedic times, Indian chanting comes out of a tradition that believes in the creative power of sound and its potential to transport us to an expanded state of awareness. The *rishis*, or ancient seers, taught that all of creation is a manifestation of the primordial sound Om. Reflected in an interpretation of the word universe—"One Song"—Om is the seed sound of all other sounds. Chanting Sanskrit often and properly produces profound spiritual and physical effects.

The uses of mantra for meditation very effective and it's relatively easy for beginners. Chanting, on the other hand, can be frightening for some people. If you feel awkward chanting on your own, use one of the many audiotapes recommended by tour instructor, or participates in a group meditation where a meditation teacher leads the chant and the students repeat it. Although chanting in Sanskrit can be powerful, reciting a meaningful prayer or affirmation in any language can be effective.

The Use of Imagery

This is the method beginners often find easy to practice. Visualizing is a good way to meditate; generally, a mediator visualizes his or her chosen deity (a god or goddess) in a clear and detailed fashion. Essentially any object is valid.

Some practitioners visualize a natural object, such as a flower or the ocean; others meditate on the chakra or energy centers in the body. In this type of meditation, you focus on the area or organ of the body corresponding to a particular chakra, imagining the particular color associated with it.

Gazing

Another divergence on the use of imagery is to maintain an open-eyed focus upon an object. This focus is referred to as Drishti, which means "View, opinion, or gaze." Again the choices available to you here are basically limitless. Candle gazing is a popular form of this method. Focusing on a flower in a vase, or a statue, or a picture of a deity are other possibilities.

Use this method with your eyes fully opened or partially closed, creating a softer, dispersed gaze. Many of the classical hatha yoga postures have gazing points, and the use of Drishti is especially emphasized in the Ashtanga style of hatha yoga. Many pranayama techniques also call for specific positioning of the eyes, such as gazing at the "Third Eye," the point between the eyebrows or at the tip of the nose.

Breathing

Using the breath as a point of meditation is yet another possibility. You can start this by actually counting the breaths as you would in pranayama practice. Ultimately, however, meditating on the breath just means purely observing the breath as it is, without changing it in any way. In this instance, the breath becomes the sole object of your meditation. You observe every distinction of the breath and each sensation it produces: how it moves in your abdomen and torso, how it feels as it moves in and out of your nose, its quality, its temperature, and so on. Though you are fully aware of all these details, you don't dwell on them or judge them in any way; you remain detached from what you're observing. What you discover is neither good nor bad; you simply allow yourself to be with the breath from moment to moment.

Breath observance is the predominant technique used by practitioners of *vipassana*, commonly referred to as "Insight" or "Mindfulness" meditation. Popularized by such renowned teachers, such as Thich Nhat Hanh, Jack Kornfield, and Jon Kabat-Zinn, this is a form a Buddhist practice. The word vipassana, which literally means "To see clearly" or "Look deeply," is also interpreted to mean "The place where the heart dwells," and reflects the premise that thought arises out of our hearts.

Physical Sensations

Another way to meditate is to watch a physical sensation. Practice this with the same degree of detail as you would when watching the breath. In this context, you will look deeply at, or penetrate a particular sensation that draws your attention, such as how hot or cool your hands feel. The increased sensitivity you gained due to your asana practice may provide you with other points of focus; for example, the strength of your spine or the suppleness you feel in your lower body. Observing a particular emotion or any specific area of discomfort is also a possibility. Whatever you choose remains your point of focus for the whole practice. You may find that observing a physical sensation can be more challenging than observing the breath. For most beginners, mantras, chants, and visualizations offer more tangible ways to replace or calm the scattered thoughts of our minds, which seem to be perpetually on sensory overload.

Meditation Postures

Meditation can easily be done in any posture; you can become fully absorbed in any activity or position of stillness. Sitting is the most commonly recommended posture in yoga practices.

Sitting

Sitting is the most recommend posture, there are several classic seated poses, but Shukhasana (Easy Cross-Legged Pose) is obviously the most basic while the more flexible mediators prefer Padmasana (Lotus Pose).

This is the best choice for beginners; it's very effective and certainly no less spiritual. The most important things are that your spine remains upright and that you feel steady and comfortable, the same two qualities necessary for performing the asana. To maximize comfort on the floor, place a cushion or folded blanket under your buttocks to elevate them and gently guide your knees down toward the floor. This helps to support the natural lumbar curve of the lower back. Some people prefer kneeling "Japanese-style." You can buy small, slanted wooden benches for this position.

Relax your arms and place your hands on your thighs or in your lap, with the palms in a relaxed position facing up or down. Roll your shoulders back and down and gently lift the chest. Keep your neck long and the chin tilted slightly downward. Depending upon which technique you are following, the eyes may be opened or closed. Breathing is natural and free.

Walking

This is a moving meditation highly recommended by many teachers; it may be an enjoyable option for you. The challenge of this form is to walk slowly and consciously, forgetting the past and aiming for the present, each step becoming your focal point. Your destination, distance, and pace all become a secondary goal. Relax your arms at your sides and move freely, coordinating your breath with your steps. For instance, you might breathe in for 3 steps and breathe out for 3 steps. If that feels awkward or difficult, just breathe freely. Although you can practice walking meditation anywhere, choose a setting you particularly love—the ocean, a favorite park, or a meadow. Remember, getting somewhere is not the issue. Rather, the complete involvement in the act of walking becomes your meditation.

Standing

Standing is another meditation practice that can be very powerful, but it is less recommended by many teachers because of stressful quality. It is often recommended for those practitioners who find that it builds physical, mental, and spiritual strength. Stand with your feet hip-to shoulder-distance apart. Knees are soft; arms rest comfortably at your sides. Check to see that the whole body is aligned in good posture: shoulders rolled back and down, chest open, neck long, head floating on top, and chin parallel to the floor. Either keep your eyes open or softly close them.

Reclining

Even though lying down is associated with relaxation, the classic Corpse Pose, Savasana, is also used for meditation. Lie down on your back with your arms at your sides, palms facing upward. Touch your heels together and allow the feet to fall away from one another, completely relaxed. Although your eyes may be opened or closed, some people find it easier to stay awake with their eyes open. A supine meditation, although more physically restful than other positions, entails a greater degree of alertness to remain awake and focused. Therefore, beginners may find it more difficult to meditate in this position without falling asleep.

The Benefits of Meditation

Research has confirmed what the yogis of ancient times already knew: Profound physiological and psychological changes take place when we meditate, causing an actual shift in the brain and the involuntary processes of the body.

This is how it works. An instrument called an electroencephalogram (EEG) records mental activity. During waking activity, when the mind constantly moves from one thought to another, the EEG registers jerky and rapid lines categorized as beta waves. When the mind calms down through meditation, the EEG shows waves that are smoother and slower and categorizes them as alpha waves. As meditation deepens, brain activity decreases further. The EEG then registers an even smoother, slower pattern of activity we call theta waves. Studies on meditators have shown decreased perspiration and a slower rate of respiration accompanied by a decrease of metabolic wastes in the bloodstream. Lower blood pressure and an enhanced immune system are further benefits noted by research studies.

Meditation is beneficial to health because it produces naturally reflects the mental and physical effects of this process. At the very least, meditation teaches you how to manage stress, reducing stress; control stress and turn it to enhance your overall physical health and emotional well-being. On a deeper level, it can add to the quality of your life by teaching you how to be fully alert, aware, and alive. In short, it helps you to understand yourself better. You are not meditating to get anything, but rather to look inwardly at yourself and let go of anything you need to let go.

Starting Your Own Meditation Practice

Yoga highly recommends a period of daily meditation. Add it to the end of your asana practice, or set aside another spare of time. You must find a time that works best for you. Don't rush yourself, don't do too much too soon; you're liable to get discouraged and stop altogether.

When and Where to Practice

It advisable you meditate at the same time and in the same place every day so as to establish consistency, choose a place that is quiet, pleasant, where you'll be undisturbed.

Normally the morning is considered the optimal time because you are less likely to be distracted by the demands of your day. Many people find that morning meditation helps them enter the day with a greater degree of composure and calmness. However, if a morning practice is not possible, try an afternoon or early evening meditation.

If you are new to yoga and meditation, you may find adding 5 or 10 minutes of meditation at the end of your asana practice enough. When meditating independently of your yoga practice, a 15 to 20 minutes time frame seems manageable for most beginners.

Posture

Choose a position that best works for you. If you prefer sitting, either on a chair or the floor, keep the spine erect and the body relaxed. Your hands should rest comfortably on your lap or thighs, with the palms up or down. If you choose to walk or stand, maintaining good posture is also important, with your arms hanging freely by your sides. When lying down, place yourself in a balanced and comfortable position with the appropriate support under your head and knees if needed.

Method

Find a method that is suitable to your point of focus. If sound suits you, create your own melody or chant, silently or audibly repeating a word or phrase if that is calming to you, such as "Peace," "Love," or "Joy."

Words of affirmations also work. it boasts the inner spirit words like "I am relaxed" or "I am calm and alert" as you breathe out. Using a tape of chants or listening to a relaxing piece of music are also options.

If you choose imagery, visualize your favorite spot in nature with your eyes closed, or gaze upon an object placed in front of you: a lighted candle, a flower, or a picture of your favorite deity.

One way to observe your breath is to count it: Breathe in for two to seven counts and breathe out for the same length of time. Then shift to simply observing the breath, noticing its own natural rhythm and its movement in your figure.

Whichever posture and method you choose, stick with them for the duration of your meditation period. Indeed, once you find what works for you, you'll want to maintain that practice indefinitely.

How Do You Know If It's Working?

At the beginning you might feel meditating annoying and uncomfortable—sitting for 20 minutes may cause your legs to fall asleep or aches, walking slowly may bring up feelings of impatience or turmoil, and reclining poses may merely make you fall asleep. Conversely, you may have some profound experiences the first few times you sit, only to spend the next few frustrating days trying to duplicate them. Relax. Meditation shouldn't cause you to feel unreasonably stressed or physically uncomfortable. If it does, reduce the length of your practice time or change your position (from walking to sitting; from sitting to standing). If that doesn't work, go back to incorporating a few minutes of meditation into your asana practice instead of holding onto a formal practice. After a few days, try returning to your normal meditation routine.

If you continue having trouble with your meditation practice, you may need to seek the guidance of an experienced teacher or the support of a group that meets regularly to meditate together. Indications of your progress, with or without a teacher or group, are feelings of mental calm and physical comfort, and the ability to be present in all your experiences.

Want to relax? Try yoga

Yoga practice is proven to help reduce stress, and the health effects stress causes to the human body. The best part is you don't need any prior experience to benefit from the practice. Whether you are at home, work or somewhere in between, yoga is always here to help you relax. We'll show you how to get started.

What You Need

You don't need anything, but yourself. If you have a yoga mat, that's great, but not necessary. A towel works, too, or you can just sit on the floor. Find a comfortable spot where you can be alone and uninterrupted for only five minutes. Depending on how your body feels, you may want to use a yoga block, blanket, or meditation cushion to place underneath your body to support your body in a comfortable seated position.

You can also take this same yoga and mindfulness practice outside for a change of scenery and influx of nature. Experiencing the vibrant colors sounds and feel of the outdoors during your yoga practice can provide a positive energy boost.

Start With Some Mindfulness

Let's start with your breath. This is a great way to slow down, become present in the moment, and connect with you:

- While sitting, allow your shoulders to relax. Extend your tailbone down and contract your stomach, which will help to straighten your back and lengthen your return from the top of your head.
- Inhale for six seconds while pushing your stomach away from your body.
- Exhale; allow your stomach to come back to your body.
- Do this four times (or more if time permits).

Now Begin

As you start yoga posture, think about yourself, self-respect, and curiosity toward yourself and your moment-to-moment experience. This will put you in the right mind space for the exercises.

1. **Relaxed Pose**: Begin in a comfortable seated position, legs crossed. Relax your feet and allow your abdomen to be in a neutral position. Think about how you are breathing; control your breathing. Feel the sensations in your body. Sit for a minute and feel the feelings that come with being unrushed, still, and internally aware.

2. **Neck Roll**: Allow your head to fall toward your chest and slowly move your head around in a full circle to the right three times and then to the left three times. Invite the feeling of letting go. Return to the relaxed pose and lift the crown of your head.

3. **Shoulder Roll**: Roll your shoulders in forwarding circular motions four times and then backward four times. When you are finished inhale, bringing your hands overhead, then placing your hands together on chest level and exhale

4. **Tabletop Position**: Slowly move onto your hands and knees, placing your wrists directly under your shoulders and your knees under your hips. Your palms should be on the floor, fingers facing forward with your weight evenly distributed on your palms. Center your head in a neutral position and soften your gaze downward.

5. **Cow Pose**: Inhale as you move your belly toward the mat. Lift your chest and look up toward the ceiling. Pull your shoulders away from your ears.

6. **Cat Pose**: Exhale and pull your stomach toward your spine and round your back toward the ceiling. Gently release the top of your head toward the floor.

7. Repeat Cat-Cow five to 10 times in an unrushed and peaceful rhythm.

8. **Downward Facing Dog**: push your toes under your feet, press your palms into the floor and lift your hips, extending your tailbone toward the ceiling. Push your heels back and slightly down toward the mat. Your heels do not have to touch the ground. Allow your head to drop so that your neck is long. Stay here for a few deep breaths.

9. **Standing Forward Bend**: Slowly move your hands to your feet and release the muscles in the neck and shoulders. Also, release the weight of your head and allow your legs to be straight.

10. **Cross Your Forearms**: Place your right hand in front of your left upper arm and weave your left arm behind your right upper arm. Press your heels into the floor and extend your tailbone up to the ceiling. Shake your head back and forth to release your neck. Stay here for at least three breaths before releasing the arms from the crossed position.

11. **Mountain**: Bend your knees, pull your stomach toward your back and roll your body up.

12. **Upward Salute**: Extend your tailbone down. Inhale here and place your hands together at chest level.

13. **Standing Forward Bend**: Slowly move your hands to your feet and release the muscles in the neck and shoulders. Also, release the weight of your head and allow your legs to be straight.

14. An additional option is to bend the knees slightly to place one palm flat on the floor or onto a block or anywhere on your leg other than your knee and raise the opposite hand over the head. Try to align the shoulders, slightly twist, and look up following the length of the extended arm. Do this on both sides.

15. **Child's Pose**: Softly come to your knees in a kneeling position. Extend your hands forward in front of you. Allow your figure to relax down and back onto your thighs. Allow space between your knees and the toes to touch. If possible, allow the buttocks to touch the heels of your feet.

Practice Yoga Anywhere

Outer from yoga class, you can do practice this wherever you may be. The time we spent commuting, changing and showering after class, even finding a yoga studio to practice away from home can be a significant (sometimes worthy) investment. Still, it also requires time, money, and possibly childcare arrangements. Cultivating a home practice can enable you to keep up with yoga even when you can't make it into a studio.

The following tips will make it easier:

Start Small: Begin with a short array, such as the one included in this guide. You may think of yoga as what you experience in an hour-long class, but your home practice maybe a few postures paired with meditation.

Ensure that you practice in a quiet place: This is very important, but where this is not possible, you could put on headphones that move well and play music from your favorite yoga playlist (below). Place your yoga mat on hardwood or cement (ideally, not carpet). If you must use a carpet, use a sturdy mat.

Try to practice at the same time every day to work it into your daily routine. It advisable you have a particular time to train, don't give up if you forget for a day or a week or even a year -- the yoga is always there for you.

Add Some Music

Music can be a motivator to get on the mat at home or in a class, even duo some yoga traditions do not encourage music. If you like to practice with music, the choices you make can help to set you in the mood. This varies widely by studio and teacher, so to get a sense of different options, yoga has several kinds of music which propels you to the feeling. This music can be used in a home practice, by yoga teachers' in-studio classes or just listened to for fun anytime:

The science of it all

Much research has been done to support the idea that yoga can reduce stress, and results have shown that yoga is a tool for stress reduction.

Yoga and Your Nervous System

One way yoga reduces stress is through regulating the nervous system, specifically the autonomic nervous system and its response to stress. You may think that yoga should focus primarily on relaxation and meditation if you want to reduce weight. Still, relaxed forms of yoga are helpful to improve your ability to return to a calm state after stress required a well-toned nervous system that is resilient. Think of it this way: If we could spend all our time in a quiet, peaceful environment, then stress would not be an issue. So changing the types of yoga, you do to include both slower and more vigorous practices can help improve our nervous system's ability to find balance and cope with stress.

Yoga and Your Genes

There is growing evidence that yoga and other mind-body mediations can alter the expression of specific genes and reduce the inflammatory response that causes disease, aging, and stress in the body.

Similarly, yoga has helped to improve the tail-end of genes, which can shorten and fray due to many factors like aging, disease, poor nutrition, smoking, and chronic stress. A study has shown that yoga can help lengthen and strengthen telomeres, which are the parts of our DNA that protect the genes from damage.

Yoga Precautions

Yoga is generally considered safe for most healthy people when practiced under the guidance of a trained instructor. On the other hand, there are some situations in which yoga might pose a risk.

It essential you see your health care provider before you start yoga if you have any of the following conditions or situations:

- A herniated disk
- Uncontrolled blood pressure
- Eye conditions, including glaucoma
- Pregnancy — although yoga is generally safe for pregnant women, certain poses should be avoided
- Severe balance problems
- A risk of blood clots
- Severe osteoporosis

You may be able to practice yoga in these situations if you take certain precautions like avoiding certain poses or stretches. If you develop symptoms, such as pain, or have concerns, see your doctor make sure you're getting benefit and not harm from yoga.

Getting Started

You can learn yoga from books and videos, but beginners usually find it helpful to learn with an instructor. Classes also offer intimacy and friendship, which are also crucial to overall well-being.

When you find a class that sounds interesting, talk with the instructor so that you know what to expect.

Questions to ask include:

- What are the instructor's qualifications? Where did he or she train, and how long has he or she been teaching?
- Does the instructor have experience working with students with your needs or health concerns? If you have a bruising knee or an aching shoulder, can the instructor help you find poses that won't provoke your condition?
- How demanding is the class? Is it suitable for beginners? Will it be easy enough to follow along if it's your first time?
- What can you expect from the class? What can you expect from the instructor? What is the aim of the course? Does it suit your needs, such as stress management or relaxation, or is it geared toward people who want to reap other benefits?

These questions enable you to know what you are expecting from the instructor.

Achieving the right balance

Every person has a different body with different abilities. You may need to modify yoga postures based on your strengths. Your instructor may be able to suggest modified poses. Choosing an instructor who is experienced and who understands your needs is essential to safely and effectively practice yoga.

Regardless of which type of yoga you practice, you don't have to do every pose. If a pose is uncomfortable or you can't hold it as long as the instructor requests, don't do it. Excellent instructors will understand and encourage you to explore, but not exceed your limits.

Chapter 8 - The Spiritual, Mental, And Self-discipline Benefits Of Yoga

Most people only understand the physical aspect of yoga, which entails stretching and attitude to agile up the body and improve posture, but there is more to yoga than this. It also has a profound impact on a person's life because of the way that it changes the mind in three unique ways. The amazing benefits of yoga practices are listed below.

Spiritual Awakening

Although yoga is not a religion, the practice can affect a person in a spiritual sense because of the seven religious laws that yoga students are taught to follow. These laws act as guides to help people find the path to inner peace through love and compassion for themselves and others. For example, one of the laws is about karma. It helps us to understand that the way that we treat other animals and humans comes back to us. So, in other words, if we act with kindness, we will receive consideration in return.

Mental Focus and Clarity

Yoga highlights the importance of regular meditation because of the way that it helps a person to keep their thoughts positive. Any time that negative thinking comes through during meditation, it is gently pushed away by refocusing on breathing and relaxation of the body. This is very important in maintaining emotional health since significant causes of stress, anxiety, and depression are the inability to see all of the proper aspects of life. So by learning to guide one's thoughts back to the present moment, these negative feelings will diminish. Other means of relaxation can also range in exercise and hot baths, which are high in conjunction with yoga.

Self-discipline and Control

Yoga helps to control one's thoughts and physiological response to surrounding stress, and a person can do more than they ever thought was possible. Yoga allows people to become more mentally and physically disciplined, so they can let go of fears or situations that have been holding them back from what they want to achieve. One way that this is done is by using a mantra during meditation. There should be a particular keyword or phrase been focused on during each session. The person repeats it aloud or in their mind. This helps to invade it into the subconscious to make success in that area happen more quickly. Yoga also teaches that if someone begins to see the world around them as a constant source of energy that they are tied to, then they can tap into that energy to be able to manifest their desires. This contributes to a change in the prevailing mentality of being stuck without hope because of self-sabotage.

Chapter 9 - Conclusion

Yoga is a subject that can be looked at intellectually, useful, and beneficial ideas imbibed. Yoga can be drunk by adopting individual attitudes that alter the nature of the samskaras. Yoga can be absorbed by living in an ashram environment. It helps us to be aware of the physical, mental, and spiritual dimensions at the same time. Yoga can be learned in a classroom environment as science, psychology or an applied subject, to provide new understanding and insight to life process, into areas where karmas are performed, into zones which shape the inner being in terms of awareness, internal development, the experience of harmony or balance, eventually culminating in the knowledge of samadhi and the fullness of wisdom, prajna.

A state of yoga can be attained when wisdom is established. This has been the vision of the seers who brought forth Satyananda yoga. This yoga is presented in the form of a lifestyle, understanding, and attitude. It is represented as an integral part of the day-to-day activities of understanding one's dharma and kartavya, obligations, and responsibilities, and trying to see the whole world as one slowly evolving and unfolding unit.

These are the components of Satyananda yoga. Many yoga masters and their schools have developed their brand of yoga. Some maters have followed and spread the path of hatha yoga while some bhakti-yoga, others jnana yoga, and kundalini yoga. Yet others have followed different trends of yoga. Satyananda yoga, which is also known as Bihar yoga, is pursuing a direction of yoga, which is trying to mold itself to the conditions of day-to-day life and by becoming part of one's life, creating a different level of understanding about the desires, inhibitions, attachments, and passions.

One of the spotlights of Satyananda yoga is practicing yoga as sadhana. To perfect yoga, one should try to develop a tyaga or renunciation. Many aspirants find that they can renounce certain things, which they may not need, but there is a tendency to cling to objects, people, and ideas with whom there is an association. Renunciation should not be isolated from the beauty of life. For those who take it to be isolated and try to be something they are not, the tyaga is a complicated process. Some people, however, do pass through this process and attain enlightenment.

If there is a need for self-expression, society provides different areas to meet those needs. Each stage of life has been given different sets of karmas and dharmas, and, in these various stages, different roles can be played. In grihastha ashrama or householder life, one can play the role of a responsible, caring, expressing one's needs, achievements, and thoughts, fulfilling whatever one wishes to attain in life. In a student's life, there is the freedom to learn, understand, imbibe, enjoy, and equip oneself with the means to succeed in life.

This is the language of the Bhagavad Gita. There has to be acceptance of the reality that is oneself, that expresses itself through the form of emotions and feelings, without attachment yet with awareness. Remaining aware of such transformations is difficult, but tyaga is a pre-condition as are acceptance and non-attachment. One has to know what one wants to attain in life, which is not just related to the world of Maya, following the human instincts of Sahara (craving), Nidra (sleep), Bhaya (fear), and Maithuna (sex). There has to be awareness. These are some of the pre-conditions of perfecting Bihar yoga.

www.ingramcontent.com/pod-product-compliance
Lightning Source LLC
Chambersburg PA
CBHW070745250726

48662CB00004B/1648